YOUR KNOWLEDGE HAS VALUE

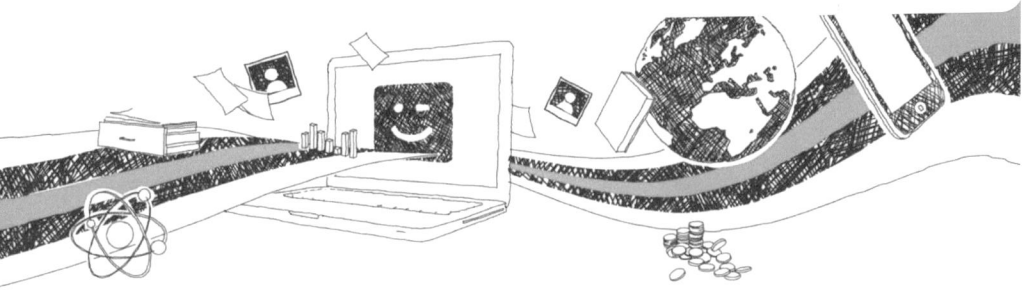

- We will publish your bachelor's and master's thesis, essays and papers

- Your own eBook and book - sold worldwide in all relevant shops

- Earn money with each sale

Upload your text at www.GRIN.com
and publish for free

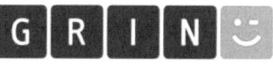

Bibliographic information published by the German National Library:

The German National Library lists this publication in the National Bibliography; detailed bibliographic data are available on the Internet at http://dnb.dnb.de .

This book is copyright material and must not be copied, reproduced, transferred, distributed, leased, licensed or publicly performed or used in any way except as specifically permitted in writing by the publishers, as allowed under the terms and conditions under which it was purchased or as strictly permitted by applicable copyright law. Any unauthorized distribution or use of this text may be a direct infringement of the author s and publisher s rights and those responsible may be liable in law accordingly.

Imprint:

Copyright © 2016 GRIN Verlag, Open Publishing GmbH
Print and binding: Books on Demand GmbH, Norderstedt Germany
ISBN: 9783668466883

This book at GRIN:

http://www.grin.com/en/e-book/368324/the-birth-control-pill-and-its-consequences-for-german-women-and-society

Nathalie Wilk

The birth control pill and its consequences for German women and society

GRIN - Your knowledge has value

Since its foundation in 1998, GRIN has specialized in publishing academic texts by students, college teachers and other academics as e-book and printed book. The website www.grin.com is an ideal platform for presenting term papers, final papers, scientific essays, dissertations and specialist books.

Visit us on the internet:

http://www.grin.com/

http://www.facebook.com/grincom

http://www.twitter.com/grin_com

Technische Universität München
Summer Term 2016
Seminar: Consumer History
Date of submission: 20.07.2016

The birth control pill and its consequences for German women and society

Table of contents

1 Introduction..3
   1.1 Research question and hypotheses..3
   1.2 Source criticism and fields of research 3

2 Historical background 4
   2.1 Birth control before the introduction of the pill (before 1961) 4
   2.2 The introduction of the pill (1961-1970s)..5
   2.3 The adoption of the pill in longterm (1970s - today) 7

3 Allocation and discussion of the results..8

4 Conclusion...10

5 References 11

1 Introduction

A tiny little pill has changed the life of many women around the world and in Germany. In 1961 the first birth control pill was introduced to the German market and after some initial difficulties established itself as the most prominent contraception method with more than 50% of women making use of it in Germany today[1]. I personally found the topic very interesting because it gave me the opportunity to research and reflect about a product I might be taking for granted today, but which in fact has come a long way and has left its marks. This paper will discuss the influence of the birth control pill on the Germany society by travelling through time and also by elaborating on the role of women throughout the process.

Furthermore some of the learning targets of the seminar will be scrutinized and later on adressed in the allocation of results:
- The influence of users on the innovation of the pill
- The appropriation of the new technology pill by consumers as part of the innovation process
- The consumption good pill as technical product that works as cultural sign

1.1 Research question and hypotheses

The interest of this paper lies in the adaption process of the pill and brings up the following question: **"How did the birth control pill influence German women and society?"**
Two hypotheses are imposed accordingly:
H1: The birth control pill transformed from a medical product to a consumption good.
H2: The pill had a massive effect on German society and the role of women.
In the following paragraphs a historical background of the development, diffusion and adaption process of the birth control pill will be provided in order to confirm or adjust the hypotheses proposed. Finally the results are allocated, taking into account hypotheses and learning targets. A conclusion rounds off the paper.

1.2 Source criticism and fields of research

The main difficulty of this paper was to find German scientific sources dealing with the topic on a purely national basis, as they were either not existing or not available via the library. Therefore other historical sources, for example materials provided by the museum for contraception in Vienna, graphs and statistics published by government institutions like the

---
[1] (Heßlig, 2011)

BzgA (Bundeszentrale für gesundheitliche Aufklärung) and BpB (Bundeszentrale für politische Bildung) or old magazine articles by „Der Spiegel" were used. When suitable US American sources were incorporated, as well. As the history of the pill started in the US the book „Disciplining Reproduction: Modernity, American Life and The Problem of Sex" by Clarke (1998) was very insightful when paying attention to the birth control movement in the US which will be adressed within the next pages. Grossmann (1998) in her book "Reforming Sex: The German Movement for Birth Control and Abortion Reform" in comparison, was describing the situation before the introduction of the pill in Germany between 1920-1950. Both the paper by Goldin and Katz (2002) as well as the one by Birdsall and Chester (1987) were talking about the impact of the pill on the economic situation of women and were used in order to describe the role of women in the long run after the introduction of the pill. Watkins (2012) in her paper added another perspective by paying attention to the technical product pill and how, according to her, it transformed from medication to a lifestyle drug.

2 Historical background

The history of the pill will be discussed in three steps. The first step explains the status quo before the introduction of the pill, how the innovation process towards its development took place and to which extent it was triggered by women. In a second step the paper focuses on the first years after the introduction of the pill and the controversial discussion which took place in society, mainly enforced by moral standards and the church. In a last step the focus is shifted to the long term adoption and influence of the birth control pill and its consequences for birth rates in Germany.

2.1 Birth control before the introduction of the pill (before 1961)

Contraception in the United States was forwarded by Margret Sanger (1879-1966), a prominent birth control acitivist. She was deeply involved in the project of achieving women's access to effective means of contraception in order to enhance female autonomy[2]. Sanger's motivation was experiencing the example of her mother who, after giving birth to eleven children and many miscarriages, died very young at the age of 40 years. And not only her mother, but almost all women of that time were suffering from the many child births and miscarriages. Their desire increased to control whether, when and with whom they have children. As men still decided on contraception and women had a huge knowledge gap concerning their body and birth control, Sanger decided to open the first birth control clinic in

---

[2] (Clarke, 1998)

the US in 1916. Soon afterwards women lined-up to get life-saving birth control information. Even though Sanger was sentenced to jail for a few times, she kept re-opening her clinic to pursue her mission to spread knowlegde about reproductive functions among women and fight for the women's right to determine wheter to bear children or not[3].

Until 1938 fundamental discoveries in the field of synthetic production of the hormones estrogen and ethinylestradiol took place in Germany and scientists working together with the pharmaceutics company Schering built the basis for advanced research. The Third Reich however stopped all further developments. Whereas the federal ban against contraception was lifted in the US in 1938, allowing condoms and diaphragms, in Germany §218 remained unaltered. The paragraph defined abortion as criminal act and any prevention or interruption of pregnancy was banned in order to foster the reproduction of the "valuable race". When breaking the law, punishments sometimes even went as far as death penalties[4].

The post war baby boom however got people and governments concerned about the growing population. In the 1950's the birth control movement transfered to a global scale. Taking into account these circumstances, a dinner party in New York in 1951 was held just in the right moment and can be regarded as the birth hour of the pill. The already mentioned activist Margaret Sanger (at this point in time already in her seventies) hosted the dinner party to which she invited Katharine McCormick, a wealthy widow and supporter of Sanger's birth control movement, and the gynocologist Gregory Pincus. During a conversation Sanger asked Pincus how much it would cost to develop a cheap and efficient contraceptive. The story ended with McCormick investing two million dollars into research which allowed Pincus to develop the first birth control pill. What's especially interesting about this story is the fact, that two women (Sanger and McCormick) were acting as drivers for the development process and hereby influencing and speeding up the innovation of the birth control pill[3].

2.2 The introduction of the pill (1961-1970s)
After the introduction of the birth control pill in the US in 1960, the pharmaceutical company Schering also introduced a contraceptive pill under the name "Anovlar" in Germany one year later on June 1st, 1961[5]. In contrast to the United States, the pill was accepted way slower due to mostly moral hazards.

---

[3] (Clarke, 1998)
[4] (Grossmann, 1998)
[5] (Museum für Verhütung und Schwangerschaftsabbruch, 2013)

In the first years the pill was only distributed to married women with children. As sex before marriage was still a tabu, contraception officially wasn't necessary for young, single women[6]. Due to this social pressure Schering advertised the pill not as contraceptive, but as a method to ease menstruation malfunction. Some gynocologist however still refused it and in 1964, 185 doctors and professors showed their protest against the pill officially in the "Ulmer Manifest". And not just doctors but also the church expressed their disapproval, which culminated in Pope Paul VI.'s Enzyklika "Humana Vitae". The pope forbid the pill for contraceptive reasons, as sex in his eyes should just have the sole reason of reproduction[5]. His strong stand divided the church by disagreement as some of the priests were of a different opinion as for example an „Der Spiegel" interview with the Jesuit priest Dr. Jakob David showed very openly[7].

The role of the woman in this period of time was quite submissive, with neither men wanting her to be independent when it came to contraception, nor the church accepting her to steer her own nature. This role however started to change slowly as it can for example be observed in an advertisement by Enovid, a pharmaceutical company: Here, Andromeda, a female figure in Greek mythology, frees herself from her chains, symbolizing the new contraceptive and the self-determination it brought to women. [5]

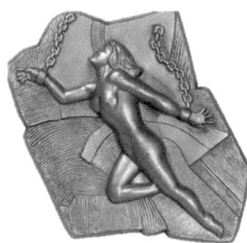

Source: Advertisement for Enovid, the first contraceptive pill [8]

Also doctors slowly lost their prior prejudices as stated by a "Der Spiegel" article from 1966: While in the beginning the pill was accused of causing cancer, those rumors were diminished through research and by magazines like "Deutsches Ärztblatt", received by every doctor in the country, showing its support towards the pill, paving the road for its broad acceptance[9].

---

[6] (M. Hentschel & Müller, 1964)
[7] (n.a., 1968) Artikel in "Der Spiegel" – Autor unbekannt
[8] (Museum für Verhütung und Schwangerschaftsabbruch, 2013):
http://en.muvs.org/contraception/c-media/enovid-badge-id2333/
[9] (n.a., 1966) Artikel in "Der Spiegel" – Autor unbekannt

2.3 The adoption of the pill in longterm (1970s - today)

The doubts and moral hazards present in the 1960s are almost forgotten today, with the pill, according to a study by BZgA, being the most frequently used contraceptive in Germany with 53% of women using it on average. Among the 18-29 year olds, it's even an impressive 72% of women who choose the method [10].

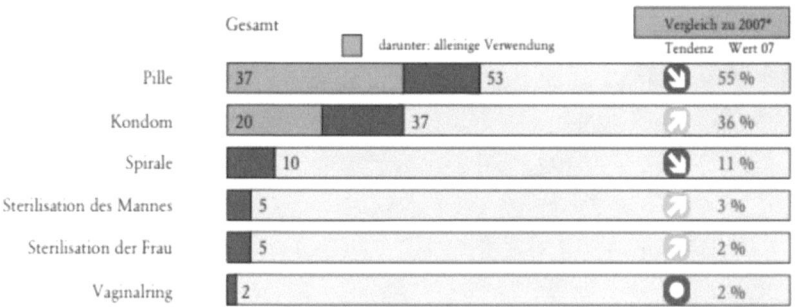

Source: BZgA Verhütungsverhalten Erwachsener[10]

The pill has found its way into our day-to-day lifes, it is social consensus to take it and to girls under 20 years it is even distributed for free[11]. Manufacturers, doctors and consumers have understood the purpose of the pill as prevention of pregnancy as a basic health care need of women. Furthermore the class of so called lifestyle drugs is increasing and one could argue that the pill belongs to this group[12].

The birth control pill is easy-to-use and very safe. It involves low health risks and few annoyances for its users, but what's even more substantial – it is female controlled. And this detail also changed the role and economic status of women[13]. Women could now delay their marriage to pursue a career: In the US an increase in female college students was noted - the pill gave women a certain planning security concerning long-term education and career investment, which couldn't be counteracted by unwanted pregnancy anymore[14]. In Germany the famous "Pillenknick" was observed. The effect was the strongest in Western Germany and decreased birth rates significantly, also confirmed by former chancellor Helmuth Schmidt who perceived both emancipation of women and the birth control pill as huge impact factors

---

[10] (Heßlig, 2011)
[11] (A. Hentschel, 2011)
[12] (Watkins, 2012)
[13] (Birdsall & Chester, 1987)
[14] (Goldin & Katz, 2002)

for the development of the German society, concerning a low birth rate as well as and an ageing population[11]. In just 10 years, from 1965-75, Germans reduced the amount of children per woman from 2,5 to 1,4 which can be observed in the following graph from Bundeszentrale für politische Bildung[15].

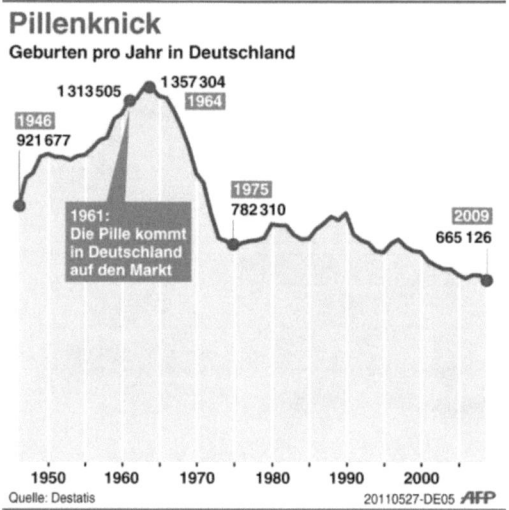

Source: Bundeszentrale für politische Bildung[15]

3 Allocation and discussion of the results

Let's bring back to memory the two hypotheses imposed in the beginning of this paper and allocate them according to the new knowledge gained:

H1: The birth control pill transformed from a medical product to a consumption good.

Throughout history, one could definitely notice a change in the perception of the pill. Thinking back to its introduction I find it very interesting to see how Schering as a manufacturer and distributor first proposed an alternative mode of consumption for the pill. Being pressured by society and moral hazard, Schering advertised the pill not as a contraceptive, but as a medication to ease menstruational disfunctions[16].

The cultural loading of the pill is still today influenced by laws and regulations, controlling its distribution and making it necessary to see a doctors in order to receive a prescription. The fact that the pill cannot be bought spontaneously at the drug store also changes the

---

[15] (Hradil & BpB, 2012)
[16] (Museum für Verhütung und Schwangerschaftsabbruch, 2013)

semiotisation of the product and might make us perceive it rather as a medical good. When talking to my mother who has been a gynocologist since 1984 however, I found out that she had noticed an increase in acceptance of the pill within society, leading to the contraceptive today being perceived rather as a necessity than a medical product. By some authors the pill gets even assigned to the product category of lifestyle drugs[17]. A clear answer to this hypothesis therefore is not possible and depends on personal and societal context, on the consumption regime involved. I personally see it rather as an everyday consumption good as already mentioned in the introduction part of this paper.

H2: The pill had a massive effect on German society and the role of women.
H2 can be confirmed more clearly. Both the effect on society and women could be proven. While helping women to gain more control and self-determination over their body, the pill also enabled them to focus on their education and career and fostered emancipation and gender equality. As a result birth rates dropped tremendously, influencing society as such, leaving Germany with independent, powerful women, but also an increasingly ageing and shrinking population.

After learning about the history and development of the pill in Germany, I also would like to reflect upon the learning targets of the seminar in this context. Interestingly users themselves were having a huge influence on the innovation process, with Margaret Sanger and Katharine McCormick acting as drivers and accelerators of the development of the pill in order to increase self-determination among younger women, fighting for the rights of the following generation. The author Oudshoorn who is focusing on co-creation of technology via users, in particular touches the role, technologies play in stabilizing particular conventions of gender, as gender is not something that we are but something we do. In the case of the pill, the technology constituted strong alignments between femininity and taking responsibility for reproduction[18].
The way users appropriate new technologies defines and shapes their cultural meaning. I think the mentioned advertisement by Enovid with the powerful woman freeing herself from her chains illustrates this process quite nicely. Whereas the pill of course had a functionality – preventing unwanted pregnancies – it's cultural meaning was really strong. By enpowering women to decide for themselves and one could even say, mechanizing their bodies (as

---

[17] (Watkins, 2012)
[18] (Oudshoorn, 1994)

discussed in class), the contraceptive symbolizes much more than just an innovative medication.

Even though the first contraception pill was developed in the US, I wouldn't speak of Americanization in this context, as also German scientist were working on a similar solution, but had to stop their work due to political reasons in the period of the Third Reich[19]. Also during our discussion in class it became clear that the birth control pill was not regarded as an American product as such, especially compared to a very culturally loaded phenonema like the Coca Cola.

4 Conclusion

By starting a journey through the history of the birth control pill, this paper aimed at clarifying the importance and meaning of the pill for both myself and the reader, as we are taking so many things for granted without further questioning their meaning. The cultural sign behind this tiny pill however is huge – enabling self-determination of women, liberating them and moving a big step towards gender equality. The paper outlined the change of the role of women through the pill as well as the change generated for society which most intensely can and will be felt today and tomorrow. Independent, self-determined women striving for higher working positions and equality in every area of life, men unsure about their role, some feeling intimidated some even threatend by strong women, but all together having dificulties to cope with them. And there's the shrinking and ageing society and the kind of challenges it will hold for our future.

---

[19] (Grossmann, 1998)

5 References

Birdsall, N., & Chester, L. A. (1987). Contraception and the Status of Women: What Is the Link? *Family Planning Perspectives, 19*(January-February 1987), 14-18.

Clarke, A. (1998). *Disciplining Reproduction: Modernity, American Life and "The Problem of Sex"*. Chigaco: University of Chicago Press.

Goldin, C., & Katz, L. F. (2002). The Power of the Pill: Oral Contraceptives and Women's Career and Marriage Decisions. *Journal of Political Economy, 110*(4), 730-770.

Grossmann, A. (1998). *Reforming Sex: The German Movement for Birth Control and Abortion Reform, 1920-1950*. Oxford: Oxford University Press.

Hentschel, A. (2011). 50 Jahre Antibaby-Pille in Deutschland

Nicht für alle leicht zu schlucken. *Süddeutsche Zeitung*. Retrieved from http://www.sueddeutsche.de/leben/jahre-antibaby-pille-in-deutschland-nicht-fuer-alle-leicht-zu-schlucken-1.1102606

Hentschel, M., & Müller, R. (1964). Antibabypillen nur für Ehefrauen? *Der Spiegel*.

Heßlig, A. (2011). *Verhütungsverhalten Erwachsener - Ergebnisse der Repräsentativbefragung*. Köln: Welpdruck, Wiehl Retrieved from http://www.forschung.sexualaufklaerung.de/fileadmin/fileadmin-forschung/pdf/BZGA-11-00988_Verhue_tungsverhalten_Erwachsener_DE_low.pdf.

Hradil, S., & BpB. (2012). Deutsche Verhältnisse - eine Sozialkunde Retrieved from http://www.bpb.de/politik/grundfragen/deutsche-verhaeltnisse-eine-sozialkunde/138003/historischer-rueckblick?p=all

Museum für Verhütung und Schwangerschaftsabbruch, W. (2013). Die Pillenstory: Eine vergessene Revolution.   Retrieved from http://de.muvs.org/topic/die-pillenstory-eine-vergessene-revolution/

n.a. (1966). Antibabypille - Nebel gelichtet. *Der Spiegel*.

n.a. (1968). Zerreißprobe in der Kirche. *Der Spiegel*.

Oudshoorn, N. (1994). *Beyond the Natural Body: An Archeology of Sex Hormones*. London: Routledge.

Watkins, E. S. (2012). How the Pill Became a Lifestyle Drug: The Pharmaceutical Industry and Birth Control in the United States Since 1960. *American Journal of Public Health, 102*(8), 1462-1472. doi:10.2105/AJPH.2012.300706

YOUR KNOWLEDGE HAS VALUE

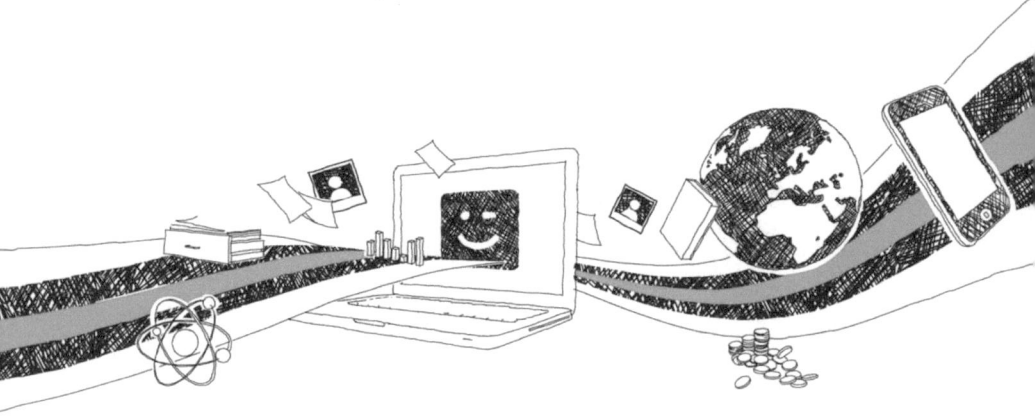

- We will publish your bachelor's and master's thesis, essays and papers

- Your own eBook and book - sold worldwide in all relevant shops

- Earn money with each sale

Upload your text at www.GRIN.com and publish for free

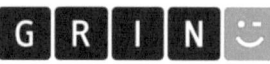